Simple Medicine

SIMPLE
MEDICINE

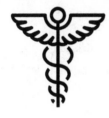

No More Google Searches

Dr. Rob Barkett Jr, MD

NEW YORK

LONDON • NASHVILLE • MELBOURNE • VANCOUVER

SIMPLE MEDICINE

No More Google Searches

Published in New York, New York, by Morgan James Publishing. Morgan James is a trademark of Morgan James, LLC. www.MorganJamesPublishing.com

Proudly distributed by Ingram Publisher Services.

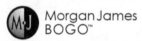

A FREE ebook edition is available for you or a friend with the purchase of this print book.

CLEARLY SIGN YOUR NAME ABOVE

Instructions to claim your free ebook edition:
1. Visit MorganJamesBOGO.com
2. Sign your name CLEARLY in the space above
3. Complete the form and submit a photo of this entire page
4. You or your friend can download the ebook to your preferred device

ISBN 9781631956492 paperback
ISBN 9781631956508 ebook
Library of Congress Control Number:
2021938727

Cover and Interior Design by:
Chris Treccani
www.3dogcreative.net

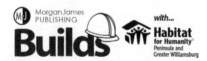

Morgan James is a proud partner of Habitat for Humanity Peninsula and Greater Williamsburg. Partners in building since 2006.

Get involved today! Visit MorganJamesPublishing.com/giving-back

Contents

Introduction

Growing up as a doctor's son in a smaller community, I was quite starry-eyed about medicine. The doctors I observed were curing the masses, loved, respected, placed upon a pedestal, wealthy, and intelligent. During medical training and after passing medical board examinations, I could diagnose and treat problems from A to Z. The problem lies in that primary care providers may see the majority of conditions once or twice in a lifetime. I have provided the most common conditions that physicians will treat daily, and they must be familiar with the atypical presentations of the common conditions. For older physicians that are stuck in their old ways, the hope is that they will see that life-changing medications and treatments are at their disposal.

Today, I am a grizzled veteran of twenty-seven years in primary care medicine. I have two target audiences: the general public who are invested in their health and primary care physicians. In the pages that follow, I will bridge old- and new-school medicine, preserving the past traditions while embracing new technologies. I will address the changing doctor-patient and doctor-doctor relationships that are quite different in this day and age.

I began practicing medicine in an autonomous situation where I could prescribe any medicine or order any study I desired. Medicine is no longer autonomous as insurance companies dictate what the physicians may do. Patients are information hungry and desire instant gratification. Patients no longer discuss their symptoms with me; they just tell me their diagnosis. Google searches have taken over their medical care. When I Google certain diseases, differential diagnoses, and medications, it is often difficult for even me to understand the explanations; it is very time-consuming, and nothing is concise. I have written this book in layman's terms and hope the general public will understand it clearly.

During patients' office visits, doctors speak in medical terms and discuss diagnostic testing and disease states as if patients actually understand what they are telling them. What I've done here is provide patients a "Cliffs Notes version" of common diseases, laboratory reviews, simplified testing, and medications that should be prescribed for common problems. Patients deserve to know what doctors are thinking and why we are prescribing certain medications and not prescribing others that are potentially harmful for them. Multiple yet equally effective screenings, tests, and treatment plans exist for every disease, including cancer. My recommendations reflect the standard of care and are cross-referenced with the American College of Physicians publication, *Medical Knowledge Self-Assessment*, Number 17.

I have grown bitter with the change in medicine, which has ruined the physician-to-physician relationships. Communication between physicians is awful as information is passed on by fax or redundant chart notes from the electronic medical record (EMR). Phone calls are almost extinct between the specialist and primary care physician. Also, EMR has changed the whole dynamic of routine office visits with patients. No longer can doctors practice medicine like the empathetic and caring Marcus Welby, MD! Since I was trained in old-school medicine and have adapted to the new technology, hospital-owned practices, hospitalists, and EMR, I believe my advice will be beneficial to the general public, medical students, residents, and young doctors. **I hope it will rattle the chain of large hospital institutions.**

Sincerely,

Robert E. Barkett Jr., MD

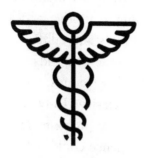

The Changing Medical World

had absolutely no desire to write a book in my lifetime. I have practiced internal medicine for the past twenty-seven years in Mansfield, Ohio and have a strong math and science background. Writing this book is a way to help my patients to the best of my ability. Over the past several years, I have noticed all the changes in the day-to-day practicing of medicine, but none of the changes have been beneficial to the doctors or to patient outcomes. I found myself constantly complaining to my wife, patients, colleagues, or anyone else who would listen to what I was saying. I felt powerless since I believe that whatever I said would probably not change anything whatsoever.

One afternoon while driving to Columbus, my wife, Melissa, was listening to another podcast by Oprah Winfrey, whom she so loves and admires. I had a revelation while Oprah was interviewing Lady Gaga, and Lady Gaga was discussing all of her wounds, trauma, and setbacks in a very raw, honest interview. Lady Gaga said if she could open up and discuss her problem, such as her abuse as a child, and her experience could help just one person, it would all be worthwhile. A lightning bolt struck my brain, and I told Melissa right then and there that I was going to write a book. She laughed, of course, since I have zero writing skills, and this was a complete shock to her.

I am very concerned over the quality of care for patients nationwide. The insurance companies, including Medicare and Medicaid, are dictating what medicines the patient may or may not have and what treatments, testing, and studies they will allow or cover. The physician-to-physician relationships and communication are starting to fail. But what is most alarming is that many patients are not receiving the standard of care for their medical conditions. This book is not intended to be a textbook but more of a reference guide to both patients and primary care providers.

My reference point comes from the new patients I see in the office from referrals from other physicians or even my current patients. Also, I am constantly reviewing medical charts as I am the medical director for both a nursing home and hospice agency. I am astonished by either their lack of care or gross neglect of the usual standard of care for treatment. I understand you can take a horse to water, but you cannot make it drink. But many patients have never been advised to have Pap smears, colonoscopies, mammograms, vaccines, spirometry, or the standard lab work. Many patients are taking way too many medications, or what we call polypharmacy, which increases the risk of drug-to-drug interactions, and some medications are contraindicated for that particular patient. I have told my colleagues many times that what I do is not brain surgery. Doctors must just take their time, keep up-to-date with the current guidelines, and have compassion for their patients. I try to treat each patient as if he or she were part of my family.

That being said, as their doctor, you cannot always be their friend. You must tell the patient the truth, convince them to do certain studies they do not want to do, and not give in to their personal request if it is not appropriate. I have angered many patients by not giving an antibiotic on their third day of a flu, refusing to give narcotics to patients with a history of alcoholism or drug addiction, refusing medications like Xanax or Ambien for the elderly, not excusing patients from work for extended periods of time for anxiety or depression, not excusing patients from jury duty, refusing handicap placards to patients who are fully capable of walking, not giving patients referrals to a specialist when it is not warranted, or scolding patients when they have not been compliant with their medications or getting their screening studies performed.

Obviously, I am not the right doctor for everyone! In the end, most patients will realize I'm only looking out for their best interests.

What I intend to do in this book is combine modern medicine guidelines with my years of experience practicing internal medicine, what is now termed "primary care medicine." What was drilled into our heads in medical school sometimes does not match up with the practice of medicine in the real world. I am going to discuss the most common reasons why patients have come to my office and, through trial and error, what I believe are the best treatment options.

The first commandment doctors learned in medical school was "Do No Harm." Academia may be critical of some of my practices, but everything I do is supported by guidelines. Unfortunately, medicine is still a practice—an art! I have failed many times, made mistakes, been short with patients, or have not discussed their problems thoroughly enough. Recognizing failures is how one becomes a better physician. I try not to make the same mistake twice. I have no disclaimers since I am in solo practice. I have no specific hospital allegiance, pharmaceutical contracts, or affiliations with any other company. I am only looking out for the best for you!

For young physicians, I'm going to give you a few tidbits I have learned through the school of hard knocks on how to interact with patients and your colleagues. A lot will sound like common sense advice. Doctors come out of residency feeling as if we can cure the world and we know everything there is about medicine! When we tell patients to do something, we optimistically expect they will do it 100 percent of the time. You see, prior to setting up our practice, we were trained in the inpatient setting where a patient's free will is not part of the equation. We were also continually supervised by our attending physician and communicated daily with our fellow residents, both of whom we knew on very personal levels. These relationships change in private practice.

The Decay of Physician-to-Physician Relationships

I was so grateful to grow up in Mansfield, Ohio in the 1970s and '80s, where I was able to witness the glory days of private medical practice. My father, Bob, was in solo practice in a town of around sixty thousand people. Internists, certainly, were the jack-of-all-trades as there were very few subspecialists, and the emergency room (ER) did not have emergency room physicians. The primary care doctors were expected to see their own patients in the ER. Primary care doctors would have to leave their private practice on a moment's notice during the day or come into the emergency room at all hours of the night. Whatever medications internists wrote or tests they ordered were actually performed.

Almost daily internists would visit their hospitalized patients, share coffee and/or breakfast with their colleagues, and consult with specialists face-to-face or by phone. I would often round with my father on weekends at the hospital , mostly to get out of my mother's hair and away from my three sisters. I knew every physician by name and the names of most of their children. I knew the nursing staff, X-ray technicians, and housekeepers. Physicians were well-respected icons of the community. Without Google searches, patients were unable to make their own diagnoses or tell the physician how they should be treated!

Doctors lived in the community they served or within twenty minutes of the hospital for their on-call duty. Doctors played prominent roles on the boards of the Chamber of Commerce, United Way, YMCA, Rotary, Kiwanis, and so on. Spouses had influential roles in the medical auxiliary and other community and philanthropic organizations. Medical families interacted with each other in dinner clubs, country clubs, and art centers while sailing, fishing, and attending theater. My mother, who is in her eighties, is still involved in a bridge club with mostly retired doctors' wives.

As of 2021, much has changed. Many physicians do not live in the communities where they practice medicine. Doctors often commute up to an hour away for their practice. It is hard to get a sense of pride or have camaraderie with your colleagues when you are not living in the same community. The real changes have evolved slowly with all the different subspecialties and technology. We have emergency room doctors who are privately owned and not even affiliated with the hospital in which they are practicing. We have specialists in the coronary care unit, critical care unit, and pediatric intensive care.

The hospitalist programs that surfaced in the 1990s have had a dramatic impact. Hospitalists are specialized doctors who work only in the hospital setting, meaning your private physician is no longer taking care of you when you are hospitalized. If a patient is sick and goes to the emergency room and the ER physician feels that the patient should be admitted to the hospital, the hospitalist is contacted, and they follow that patient throughout their hospital stay. The primary care physician no longer has that day-to-day relationship and friendship with his colleagues in the inpatient setting.

What is most disturbing is that our hospitalists do not communicate with me about my patients' admissions to the hospital or their hospital stays. A discharge summary will be faxed to my office upon their release. Our hospital administrators have tried multiple times to rectify this situation with specialized meetings amongst the physicians on improving communication, to no avail. We've suggested personal phone calls on admission and/or change in patient status. This communication could take thirty seconds, but it has not happened more than a handful of times in twenty years. When you do not have personal conversations with other physicians, it is difficult to develop any type of relationship or trust. Faxing data from the EMR—electronic medical record—is not what is best for our patients or for doctor-to-doctor relationships to grow.

I do not want to criticize only the hospitalists, as other specialists in the hospital setting are just as guilty of poor communication skills. The majority of my colleagues are awesome, know what I expect, and call me with patient changes and updates when necessary. The problem lies mostly with the younger generation of physicians who have grown up in the era of advanced technology. When I meet a physician or subspecialist to whom I may refer patients, I tell them to please give me a call anytime about my patient's status. But there have been many times my patients may have had open-heart surgery, an emergency colectomy or appendectomy, been critical in the ICU, or transferred to another hospital without my knowledge. Those physicians who did not reach out to me will attest that our next conversations were not very pleasant.

This never would have happened twenty years ago when physician relationships were stronger and experienced better communication with personal phone calls rather than with emails, texts, and faxes. In fairness, the same poor communication occurs when my patients are transferred to the Cleveland Clinic, University Hospital, or Ohio State University. One would think it would be protocol to have that particular specialist caring for my patient give the primary care provider—the quarterback of the medical team with all of the prior knowledge of the patient—a phone call. This rarely happens. Riverside Methodist Hospital is the exception as I always receive a phone call, often when my patient is still lying on the catheterization table! Thank you!

Know Your Patients

I love primary care medicine because it allows me to take care of generations of families—uncles, aunts, cousins, etc.

For 90 to 95 percent of my patients, this is a wonderful experience. Patients take their medications, follow up on a routine basis, and perform their preventive screening studies and vaccines. My care for them allows me to build a lifelong friendship. It's the minority of patients that test my nerves. No matter what I do or how much time I spend with them in the office or after hours, some patients will never be satisfied. They will call my staff on a weekly, sometimes daily, basis and complain about me, their bills, the medications, or the side effects—or are just very needy. This is still OK, and, as I said, I try to treat each patient like family. What family does not have a relative with a few personality quirks? We try to find a middle ground where everyone is somewhat satisfied.

Even in this age of a computer-driven medical system, the EMR, doctors must resist typing on the computer during the entire medical exam. I attempt as much eye contact as possible. Before each visit, I prepare to enter the room. I review old records, medications, and labs or studies that were recently performed. Patients appreciate that I have reviewed all of the prior testing and am familiar with what occurred on their previous visit. I prepare the encounter on the EMR to satisfy all requirements for a visit as much as possible prior to the exam. Insurance companies require doctors to check a thousand boxes for each exam so the doctor can actually properly bill the patient. At times, I feel more like a secretary than a physician. This is a source of much frustration for me!

As doctors, we must learn patience. No matter how far behind schedule, fatigued, sick, or edgy we are, we should treat each patient as if he or she is the only patient we have that day. Always attempt to talk about their family, personal interests, and activities before talking about medicine. When you do get down to the medical business and ask what their problem is or how they're feeling, please let them speak uninterrupted for at least two minutes. Try to resist the temptation to interrupt or redirect the conversation. If anyone knows how to do this consistently, please tell me, as I fail at this every day! As we were taught in medical school, if we listen, patients will almost always give us the diagnosis.

After being in practice for several years, I was able to get to know my patients' personality nuances and expectations and how to deal with their medical problems. When entering the exam room, I already have reviewed the reason for the patient's visit because one of my nurses has gathered this information. I can tell 90 percent of the time by the patient's body language if this patient is really sick and will require medication or further evaluation for their illness or will only require reassurance that they will be OK. Doctors must get their heads out of the computer and observe the patient as a whole. If a patient is telling you they have "ten-out-of-ten" chest, abdominal, or back pain, and they are smiling and appear to be in no acute distress, a lightbulb should go off in your head. Every patient is different. Even when a patient comes to the office on a weekly basis for some ailment, we still must take each session seriously.

As with the boy who cried wolf, we cannot jump to conclusions until we go over our usual process and checklist. Never be afraid to ask your staff's opinion since they probably know the patient better than you do. You should order the necessary testing as you see fit. Generally, most patients just need reassurance that they will be fine and are not going to die anytime soon, and this will ease their minds. I try to reiterate several times to patients that they should always call if the problem persists.

In the opposite scenario, there are patients who will not say anything, even if they should have a mouthful to communicate. When a patient comes to see me because his spouse, employer, or friend told him to, I am hyper-alert to what they have to say. Often, they underplay what is going on and tell me it's simply what happens when you get older. My interest is always peaked when my rarely-seen patient calls in for an appointment that is not for their insurance-required yearly wellness exam. The physician should always assume the worst-case scenario for the patient and go from there. I observe their facial features, tone of voice, and cold, clammy, or warm handshake, before even asking any questions.

Staff

If a physician joins an established practice or hospital-owned group, they do not have the luxury of choosing their staff. You will soon realize that a good staff is worth its weight in gold. They are the first to see your patients, set the tone, make initial assessments, and ascertain the degree of severity for the office visit. The staff represents the physician and is responsible for making the appointments, returning phone calls and emails, collecting the money, reviewing prior authorizations for medications and studies, and explaining in layman's terms what the doctor has advised the patient. I'd like to explain how each team member functions and how we are working together in my practice.

Receptionists give the first impression of the medical office as patients enter the door. My wife, Melissa, functions as my practice manager/receptionist and she or my nurses personally answer each and every phone call. We do not use automated recordings or texts to confirm appointments, as I believe it is one of the most infuriating devices I deal with as a customer. How many times do you call your doctor, pharmacy, restaurant, or even retail store and find yourself being prompted to punch ten different buttons only to be placed on hold for an indefinite time—and then the call is dropped? Shower, rinse, and repeat the same process every time.

Melissa has a wonderful smile and contagious enthusiasm and personality. She wakes up smiling and in a good mood every day, even while putting up with me! Melissa welcomes each patient, signs them in, requests the co-pay, and has personal conversations with each patient. A patient may be having a bad day and come up to the desk complaining that it is taking too long to be seen, forgot the co-pay, or simply want to chat. Melissa is the warm and fuzzy to my sometimes abrupt and prickly.

In this day and age of insurance companies, with different co-pays and payment set-ups, collecting money is a thankless job. It is imperative that we collect our co-pays on the day of appointments, or we can be out thousands of dollars. Last year, we had around 6,500 patient visits. If we wrote off ten dollars for every patient, it would add up quickly. A medical practice is, after all, still a business. Melissa works closely with our billing specialist and checks every claim before it is submitted to the insurance company. When the patients' visits are over, Melissa is the last staff member to see them before they leave, and her empathy for our patients is off the charts. She schedules them for other tests, consultations, and any follow-up visit to our office. She gets to know each patient on a personal basis just like the nurses.

Nurses

Amy and Aby are both LPNs, and they are integral to the running of my office practice. They wear multiple hats on any given day. Sometimes, they may be more of a receptionist, answering phone calls, making appointments, explaining medical treatments and medications, and developing a special friendship with the patients. My nurses check vital signs, such as blood pressure, heart rate, and respirations, and get each patient's weight, much to their dismay. They enter all of the information into the EMR, including the reason for the patient's visit. Nurses will remind me of a patient's family members' problems or dilemmas or even their kids' or pets' names. Most important to me is the triage of the severity of the problem and what their initial assessment entails. Nurses alert me if the patient may be angry, sad, or joyous or what particular events are going on in their life.

After every patient visit, I discuss with the nurse what our game plan is. They will obtain lab work; perform spirometry, an EKG, event recorders; flush ears or prepare the patient for a cardiac stress test. They schedule testing for the patient. What I treasure most is their explanation to the patients of my diagnoses and what tests I have ordered. Sometimes, after my discussions with patients, I believe all they hear is "blah, blah, blah." Perhaps I have shocked them and their minds go elsewhere. My nurses have a tremendous way of communicating what I have said and may have meant. If a doctor ever states he is looking for cancer or some other disease, it is difficult for patients to stay focused. This mindlessness has happened to me when I've been a patient. I will go home; Melissa asks me what the doctor said, and I will say I have no idea except that surgery is next Wednesday.

Since doctors are working with nurses so closely on a daily basis concerning patients' lives, there can be tension. Thank goodness we've worked together many years, and we know each other's different moods, reactions, and personality traits. The nurses may offset this tension with jokes or sarcasm or give me some space for a few moments. Their skill in interpreting my answers to them and translating this for the patients is amazing. I trust my nurses' judgments implicitly. Daily, they review my responses and answers to test results and even question me if they feel I may have overlooked something or confirm that my medical evaluation is correct.

Billing Department

Can you go to a restaurant, eat, and leave without paying? Can you go to Kroger, Best Buy, or Macy's and buy items without leaving any money? No, of course not! In this day and age of insurance, co-pays, deductibles, and EOBs (explanations of benefits), one needs a PhD to understand it all, both as a patient and as a physician. Most patients have deductibles in the thousands of dollars and are well aware they may never hit their deductible and be paying cash all year.

After much pressure from the federal government, we instituted the EMR in 2011. Learning the new system hastened the retirement of one of our nurses, who had been performing billing in-house for many years. Outsourcing to a billing company costs between 4 and 8 percent of all receivables. Since billing companies receive more money if they collect more money owed to the office, I figured they would do their job and know what they were doing. I was dead wrong. After two years and two different billing companies, I was barely able to make payroll, and we were becoming delinquent on our other bills. Even some of our patients were telling us they had not been billed for over a year.

Thank goodness we found Darlene! We saw her ad on Indeed, interviewed her, and I actually talked to references this time. Within weeks, Darlene opened Pandora's box and found error after error or just plain laziness with the other billing companies. For example, if a visit is not properly coded, the insurance company will reject the claim, and it must be resubmitted within their particular time frame. Because this was not followed up on properly, we lost thousands of dollars in reimbursements. After six months of Darlene's diligent work, we were back on our feet again. And, thankfully, due to the long-term relationships with our patients, most of them were willing to pay their outstanding balances, even though they had not been billed in a timely manner.

Doctors are never taught how to run a practice, let alone learn the financial aspects of doing it properly. Doctors are taught to take as good care of our patients as we possibly can, so it is imperative to get the best office staff to support the business so we physicians can concentrate on what we do best.

The Office Experience

The office experience is nerve-wracking, whether it is your first visit or one-hundredth visit to your doctor. Fear of the unknown is consuming. Multiple healthy patients have told me that by the time they enter our parking lot, their hearts have started racing, their blood pressure has risen, and their minds have wandered. Patients check in, pay their co-pay, and give their insurance information, and then they wait for a variable amount of time. The patient's name is called and vital signs are obtained, and the patient is placed in the examination room only to wait for another unknown amount of time. We try not to overbook our schedule, be as punctual as possible, and apologize to patients if delays occur.

Obviously, in my occupation, emergencies and other time-takers happen frequently, such as flu epidemics or complicated patients who cause me to run behind schedule. I try to remember the patient's time is just as valuable as mine, so I do everything possible to be on time. Most people will understand if running behind is unusual or happens only on occasion. Sometimes, doctors must be a patient themselves to appreciate how all this works in real life. I have been a patient and suffered from white-coat hypertension and the usual anxieties, but the worst part is waiting. In our profession, being punctual all of the time is likely impossible, but we have to do our best.

Since our patients are going to wait, we try to make the waiting room a pleasant experience. You can have a TV or music. We use Sonos, which is wonderful. Sonos runs off Wi-Fi. We play all genres of music plus seasonal favorites. A broad selection of magazines is a must. We offer *Time, People, Sports Illustrated, Better Homes & Gardens, Essence, Living with Martha Stewart*, and *Popular Me-*

chanics—something for everyone. Every three months, I go through the magazine rack to keep them current. We always have *Highlights* to entertain the kids.

You have only one chance to make a first impression! I always try to look professional with my clothing, grooming, and overall physical appearance. As primary care providers working only in the outpatient setting, there is no reason to wear scrubs, tennis shoes, or sandals. I realize dress codes have become more casual throughout the country, but a necktie, dress shirt, dresses, skirts, or pantsuits should be mandatory. Patients observe what I am wearing, and often, it becomes a topic of conversation. When I do not wear a tie, I usually go without socks with penny loafers, even during the winter. When wearing socks, I love Happy Socks, which are pretty flamboyant. I wear special socks and ties for all of the different holidays. Patients often tease or compliment me, but they are an icebreaker and tension reliever. I enjoy the banter, and it usually leads to some interesting conversations.

I believe it is imperative that doctors are well-groomed and remain in good physical shape. You must retain your individuality with your hair, glasses, and clothes. Your hair can be short, long, or styled as well as having a groomed beard. For some reason, people seem a little smarter when they are well-groomed. One of my pet peeves is morbidly obese physicians. You do not need to be a vegetarian or tri-athlete, but remaining in decent shape is the least you can do. How can doctors tell patients to eat healthy, exercise, and lose weight if the doctors themselves do not do those things? I would laugh if my three-hundred-pound doctor told me to follow a two-thousand-calorie, low-fat diet and exercise three hours a week. I would tell him to look in the mirror and explain to me why he could not follow his own advice! We must practice what we preach.

Electronic Medical Records

EMR, or electronic medical records, is the biggest evil I have encountered in primary care medicine over my twenty-seven years of private practice. I often feel like a robotic data entry clerk, punching a keyboard for certain measures the powers that be want me to punch. If I don't meet these measures, my practice can be penalized financially. I do not believe EMR has improved patient care or outcomes. It was pushed down doctors' throats during the Obama administration way before it was perfected. I'm not sure how much input was received from the medical community on how the software should be structured to make medical sense. EMR is still not close to performing the functions it was meant to do. There are multiple different EMRs, and the EMRs don't communicate with each other. Ultimately, this was the original purpose: to solve many problems with patient care that could be improved with integration.

For example, many medical EMR programs cannot even communicate with an affiliated hospital a quarter of a mile away. If my patient is admitted to the hospital, I can only view their labs and testing performed while they are in the emergency room. I cannot see any consultations or updates of their care during their hospital stay. Since hospitalists rarely call or notify the patient's primary doctor, I doubt they would take the time to check the EMR even if the systems communicated together. EMR is supposed to be a paperless system, but I believe redwood trees must be chopped down daily for the superfluous paper I receive through the fax machine every day. I counted twelve papers for an echocardiogram result the other day. All I require is the conclusion of the results on one page.

The most confusing part is trying to read different EMR reports from a specialist's consultations. A lot of data is included—most of which I already know—and it is like trying to find Waldo to figure out what that doctor is thinking and what the plan is. This is 1000 percent worse than when doctors dictated reports in one paragraph to each other. We could hit on the highlights and give a formalized plan of action. Daily, my trash bin is loaded with wasted paper and useless information. To be fair, the only portion of my own medical record that is sensible to me is the impression and plan where I type in the information. I could dictate a patient visit in about thirty seconds in the past, but now, it takes me about four minutes to put in all the data for today's patient. I hope people feel my frustration with modern technology.

EMR's advantage is that all the information is on one screen—although I must open twenty different screens to see what I need. Medications, immunizations, past surgeries, allergies, and cancer screenings are available with the click of a button, which is awesome. One distinct advantage from the past is that prescriptions are now sent electronically, so no longer does the pharmacist have to decipher my poor handwriting. I can e-prescribe directly to the local pharmacy or the mail-away program in an efficient manner.

The Examination

When I enter the examination room, I greet each patient by looking them in the eye and, until the coronavirus pandemic, firmly shaking hands. No matter how busy the day is or how frazzled or behind schedule I am, I attempt to make the patient feel as if they are the only patient I have for the entire day. I maintain eye contact as much as possible despite having to constantly enter data into the EMR, which makes it nearly impossible. I can judge so much by the demeanor, appearance, and body language of the patient, and this greatly helps with the diagnosis. Of course, it gets much easier when I have been seeing that particular patient for years. Chairs are arranged so we are looking face-to-face.

Most visits last around ten minutes, and I like to discuss personal matters at the start of each examination. I get to know the patient's family, coworkers, friends, pets, and hobbies. I readdress why the patient is here for the visit, either as a follow-up appointment or a new problem. Next is the tricky part. In medical school, we were taught to ask an open-ended question and allow the patient to speak for two minutes uninterrupted. As stated before, I am awful at this. I know I sometimes interrupt the patient and redirect their stories too much. One of the best pieces of advice I received early on was this: The patient will give me the diagnosis if I just listen.

After a review of systems, the physical exam is next. Every doctor will have his or her own routine, and I believe you must follow that routine religiously with each patient. It may seem mundane at times, but it will save lives. I begin with the head and neck examination. I'll never forget the perfectly healthy male with no complaints. As I swiped along the supraclavicular area, I found a hard, non-tender lymph node that turned out to be squamous cell carcinoma. He was eternally grateful!

Then I perform a heart, lung, and abdominal exam, and I always check for swelling (edema). If the patient comes in for a particular problem, I focus on that problem only in addition to the general exam. Patients, if a physician does not put a stethoscope on your chest or do any examination during your visit, I would suggest you find another physician. I can count too many occasions when I have heard an irregular heart rhythm that turned out to be atrial fibrillation in asymptomatic patients. Physicians, if you are examining a breast, pelvic region, or rectum of a patient of the opposite sex, you should always have a nurse as a chaperone. Never invite a potential problem that is preventable.

Once the exam has concluded, I discuss my diagnosis and treatment as plainly as I can—or what we call layman's terms. If it is complicated or bad news, I will invite the patient's significant other or family member into the room if they are in the near vicinity. I try to repeat what I say at least twice.

With medication changes, I will write down what medication will be discontinued and what the new medications are going to be and how they should be used. I write down the vaccinations I have recommended for the patient to receive at the pharmacy.

During the entire process, I realize I am spending too much time plugging information into the EMR. I apologize a lot, but this is just the way it is in modern-day medicine. When patients have explained their stories, I will speak out loud the words I'm typing. I remember the *Seinfeld* episode when Elaine goes to the doctor and freaks out because she doesn't know what he is writing down. Then she gets Kramer to break into the doctor's office to steal the medical record!

If I find an abnormality in the examination, I will stop and enter it into the EMR. I know my limitations and can no longer multitask, so I feel obligated to finish the patient note before I leave the room. I will explain to the patient which tests, laboratory work, or consultations I plan to have and when their next visit will be scheduled. I advise that if the current problem does not get any better, they should call back to the office for further evaluation. With all my good advice and intentions to others, I know I probably fail every day, and some patients may feel shortchanged. All I can do is the best I can!

FYI for patients: If you call your primary care physician for a particular problem that day, doctors will focus on that problem. Insurance companies, Medicare, and Medicaid advise this practice and will only reimburse for today's chief complaint. Plus time has been allotted only for that problem. Many patients who do not see me on a regular basis but call in to be seen on a particular day for a sore throat will bring a laundry list of questions. Do not get mad if the doctor understands your concerns but asks you to reschedule another appointment to address all of the other problems.

Honesty

Honesty seems simple, but it is often difficult to navigate through. As trained physicians, we should have all of the answers to all of the questions and diagnoses. More important than what we know is to know what we do not know. Do not fake it! It is OK to say I am not sure or I have no idea. I'll explain what I think is going on and what I am going to do to figure out the problem. When I still cannot pinpoint the diagnosis, I consult the specialists who have our backs. Patients definitely appreciate this approach.

When I am dealing with a difficult diagnosis or prognosis, I try not to candy-coat my explanation to the patient. Every physician will have their own style, but I go with my gut instinct and try to explain to the patient the worst- and best-case scenarios. I may need other studies or biopsies to pinpoint the diagnosis, but the patient has the right to know what I am thinking. I hate to scare patients, and I will tell them I'm hoping for the best.

Part of honesty is sticking to your guns. Throughout your years in practice, you develop great relationships and friends. Many patients will become your golfing, tennis, cycling, card playing, or dinner club friends. This can be a challenge at times. The relationship between a physician and patient is really more of a parent-child relationship when the patient is in the office. Physicians must not let emotions become part of the equation while making medical decisions. Your most and least favorite patient should be treated in the exact same manner. If they demand antibiotics, Xanax, sleeping pills, narcotics, or Viagra but are not appropriate candidates, say no and no again. That is why the American Medical Association frowns upon doctors taking care of their own family members.

Telling patients the truth can appear mean and abrupt. If the body mass index (BMI) is greater than thirty-one, the patient is obese. If the BMI is greater than forty, the patient is morbidly obese. A stern conversation about the complications of obesity is warranted. If the patient is a smoker and you ask the patient why they are trying to kill themselves, they will give you a weird look. A detailed explanation of the pros and cons of smoking cessation will ensue. I do not believe all patients need to like their physicians, but they should respect them. This was confirmed by the Press Gainey survey. The survey asked patients to rate their doctors and their overall experiences. The final analysis revealed an inverse relationship between patient satisfaction and patient overall health outcomes. This means the more that a patient liked their doctor, the worse the outcome that patient had. Physicians were probably giving in to patients' demands, but patients then had more severe medical outcomes. Doctors who hold their ground will definitely anger some patients, but the patients will have better health outcomes!

As an example, I have always told my patients I do not care about a surgeon's personality or bedside manner; all I care about is the skill of their hands and the complication rate. I've known or heard of physicians whose patients absolutely loved them even though they could not perform a simple operation on a patient without complications. Doctors, you have to practice medicine the way you were trained, and you must make decisions for your patients' good.

Follow-Up Care and Consultations

After the patient has left the office, the nurses make a list of the studies requested and lab work that were performed. Our practice manager checks that all tests have been ordered and all referrals have been made prior to submitting the daily charges to the billing company. Days later, our nurses double-check to ensure we did not overlook any problems and that all studies were performed and evaluated. We tell the patient no news is good news on their test results or to check the patient portal on the EMR for results or call the office back in several days. New insurance requirements stipulate that any patients admitted to the hospital must follow up with their primary care provider in one or two weeks, depending on the severity of the disease. Follow-up visits have been proven to decrease hospital readmission.

I believe one of the most important responsibilities as a primary care provider is to choose the appropriate subspecialist for a consultation when required. Subspecialists are vital to my practice and patient outcomes. I refer only to doctors I would go to myself. Not all subspecialists are created equal. I rely on my professional relationship, past experiences, reputation, and patient outcomes when determining whom I consult. I demand my patients be seen in a timely manner, be treated with respect, and expect superior outcomes and few complications. I desire to be notified in a personal manner with a phone call if the problem is serious or life-threatening or in a personal letter—and not the EMR transmission. I regard the subspecialist as a representation and reflection of me. If the patient sees a nurse practitioner or a physician's assistant after waiting two months to get in for a visit with the subspecialist, I consider this a slap in the face. If patients are not treated respectfully or with the quality of care I expect, I will have problems with the specialist. I will discuss it with them right away in a phone call. If problems persist, we can always find another quality provider.

I am an independent provider with no specific hospital affiliation other than courtesy affiliation. I choose to remain independent so I can send my patients anywhere in the state where I feel it is best for them to go. Hospital-owned primary care physicians do not have that flexibility; they are encouraged to refer to their own hospital affiliation.

As stated, all doctors are not created equal. Not everyone can be a Tiger Woods or LeBron James of their specialty. When I was approached to join a hospital-owned practice, I was offered 15 to 20 percent more money with the understanding I would keep all consultations in-house. One can probably refer to outside institutions, but it is surely frowned upon. I have had patients leave my practice because I refused a referral to a particular physician of their choosing. Again, it is about being honest, and this allows me to sleep better at night. I have never liked losing patients, but as the saying goes, you cannot have the inmates running the asylum. I am only looking out for their best interests.

New subspecialists move to our area frequently. The hospital has been very good about bringing these doctors to my office for face-to-face visits. As I only work in outpatient medicine and I do not take care of my patients while they are hospitalized, this is the only way I get to know these doctors. I like to place a name with a face, check their medical background and residency training, and find out the reasons why they are coming to our area. I observe their personality to see how they may interact with my patients. I am sometimes suspicious when a physician in their fifties or older moves to our little town after having an established practice elsewhere. If it's for family or something else reasonable, I will give them a pass, let them get their feet wet, and consult them if needed.

As an example, our local hospital often transferred patients to Columbus for a gastrointestinal (GI) bleed or a stone in the bile duct. A GI specialist moved to Mansfield from California with no family in the area. He specialized in ERCP, which extracts stones from the bile duct. He came to my office for an introduction, and I was happy that ERCP could now be performed in our area without transferring patients out of town. But I was suspicious as to why he was really here. One month later, my patient was in the emergency room with the problem he specialized in. The ER transferred my patient to Columbus because this new specialist refused to see the patient in the emergency room. Soon after, I tried to schedule another patient for an acute situation, and he could not see that patient for two weeks. I was as mad as a hornet, and needless to say, I never referred to that doctor again. The hospital did see the doctor's shortcomings and fired him. Since that incident, when a new physician moves to our area, I try to contact another doctor who may know a physician from past interactions to get an honest opinion. When all is said and done, it is all about a patient's outcomes.

Reality with Patients

I have thoroughly enjoyed my job as a physician and the relationships I have made with my patients throughout the years. Over 95 percent of the patients are a joy to work with as they take personal ownership of their health and remain compliant with their healthcare. Some patients are more of a challenge and require more reassurance and sometimes hand-holding. Some patients are just plain difficult to deal with, and I realize I will never satisfy their expectations.

As an example, early in my career, I saw a new patient for a physical, and within minutes, she told me she would see me for the simple things but for anything more complicated she wanted to be referred to Riverside Hospital in Columbus sixty miles away. I had just finished my residency at Riverside and had recently been board-certified in Internal Medicine. She was well aware of this since she had done her homework on me. When I moved from the big city to the small town, I guess I must've lost a few marbles along the way.

Early in my career, I was crushed when a patient left my practice. The reality is that patients leave a medical practice for many reasons other than death, moving out of town, or changing insurances. I try to make a positive out of the negative situation and understand how I could've been a better doctor for that patient. A doctor once told my father in his early years of medicine that you really never know who your patient is until you sign their death certificate!

Internet

Patients telling me they researched their problems online and then providing their own diagnosis used to make my hair stand on end! But in this age of instant gratification, knowledge, and access to information, I've learned to embrace the internet. The internet has challenged me to stay current on all the new medications, holistic care, and herbal remedies and refresh my memory on all day-to-day common medicine.

When patients research their ailments, it shows me they are concerned with their own healthcare. Since everything they read on the internet is true—ha ha—I must interpret what they have read. The overwhelming majority of the time, patients work themselves into a frenzy and believe they are dying. I reassure them they will be fine, and that peace of mind is a wonderful thing.

I have an example and a cute story from one of my patients. My patient was an educated person and had a new medical problem. He was worried sick, and his Google search identified a rare disease he had acquired. I explained this was probably not the case, and a simple test confirmed a diagnosis. Luckily, I was correct, and the patient was quite relieved. On his next visit, he brought me a poster that read: "Do not confuse my Google search with your medical degree!" We hung the sign in the front office and still get many laughs and comments from the quote.

Urgent Care

Maybe I'm just getting old and grumpy and set in my ways, but I have a love-hate relationship with urgent care facilities and emergency rooms. I somewhat distrust major health systems and their ability to balance medical care for all people and making the big bucks. I realize many patients will use urgent care and emergency rooms for their primary care services. I've often been told that folks have called their doctors but could not be seen in their offices for several weeks, so they went to urgent care. Quality of care may be jeopardized when these facilities are being run by nurse practitioners (NPs) or physician's assistants (PAs). These providers do not have relationships with the patients, and I have observed multiple unnecessary lab work, X-rays, and CT scan orders on a daily basis. When unnecessary testing is performed, I believe providers in these facilities order these tests to avoid potential problems. Everyone is afraid of being sued.

Ten years ago in Mansfield, we had one emergency room at MedCentral, now called OhioHealth. Urgent care facilities were almost nonexistent. OhioHealth has since opened an urgent care center and an emergency care center satellite. Avita Health System has now been around for the last ten years, and they have their own emergency room and two urgent care facilities. University Hospitals from Cleveland just opened a brand new urgent care in 2020. There are two free-standing, urgent care centers without hospital affiliation. Akron City Children's Hospital also has an urgent care center. Mansfield has been devastated by the shutdown of Westinghouse, Tappan, and General Motors and by the downsizing of other big industries and has lost more than ten thousand residents over the last few years. Our current population is around forty-four thousand people, but service extends to other surrounding smaller cities. Cleveland, Columbus, and Akron are just over one hour away. Are two emergency rooms and seven urgent care centers in a declining population really needed, or am I missing something?

In contrast, Mansfield has had a primary care physician shortage over the past thirty years, and this is predicted to get worse here and nationwide over the next ten years. You cannot just start graduating more medical doctors, so hospitals have decided that NPs and PAs are the next best option. With the number of new emergency rooms, urgent care centers, and hospital-owned primary care practices, the number of NPs and PAs has grown exponentially.

One must think about the differences in training and the pedigree required to be accepted into medical school versus NP/PA school. Medical school applicants must have a four-year bachelor's degree. When I applied to Thomas Jefferson Medical School, they received more than 10,000 applicants and accepted 228 medical students. I am guessing each applicant must have had a high grade-point average, many extracurricular activities, volunteer experience, and an adequate MCAT score. How medical schools make their decisions for acceptance must be very difficult and is anyone's guess.

Medical school is four years long with two years extensively in the classroom and two years doing rotations in most fields of medicine. I know this regimen is now integrated these days. After medical school, internal medicine and family practice residencies require three more years of training.

During my residency at Riverside Hospital, we worked twelve-hour days and every fourth day, we were on call, meaning we were at the hospital for thirty-six straight hours. We did not work Sundays unless we were on-call. We were exposed to every disease possible time and time again. Again, times have changed and residents are restrict-ed to only working sixteen hours maximum per day. My old-school ethics make me scratch my head with these new regulations! Unfortunately, I do not have personal experi-ence with NP/PA school. NPs require a four-year degree in nursing (at a minimum) and two years in an NP program. PAs require a four-year bachelor's degree and two years in a PA program. I do not know the difference in the number of total hours required for medical school versus NP/PA school, but it is significant. This reminds me of when a pa-tient asks how I know what her problem is. I state it is Aunt Minnie: "If it looks like Aunt Minnie, then it's your Aunt Minnie." Experience and training are everything.

When I hear that patients have a primary care physi-cian and it will take weeks to get an office visit, I think this is appalling. I do not care if a doctor is solo or in a group practice; it is the doctor's responsibility and obligation to see their patients in a timely fashion. My staff will triage the patient's call and complaints. If the patient is sick, they will be seen either that day or the next day, depending upon the circumstance. Sometimes, a patient who comes to the office does not agree with my advice and goes to the urgent care or emergency room anyway. Doctors cannot work 24/7, so urgent care/emergency room care is a great compliment for after-hours, weekends, and true emergencies.

As an athlete, I have learned more from the losses than the victories. I may play a nice round of golf and have sixty-nine good shots and then complain and moan about the three-putts I had or a stubbed chip shot. That probably symbolizes my thoughts on treatment and care at the urgent care/ER. They do a great job the majority of the time, but other times, I am just astonished. Z-Paks must be the most amazing antibiotic ever created. I have seen it written by urgent care providers for ear wax, one-day-old colds, a two-day history of diarrhea, and a hangnail! I have patients claim a complete resolution of a cough after only one dose. Patients may be seen for a sinus infection or bronchitis and will be given blood tests, chest X-rays, and CT scans needlessly. Fall down and hit your shoulder and you will get a CT scan of your head, neck, and entire back. I have to sell my firstborn child to get insurance to pay for a CT scan from my office.

My nurses ask why I become so perturbed when unnecessary tests are performed or why I will not order a certain study a patient requests. My answer is that it's not good medicine. Unnecessary medical testing does not cost me anything so maybe I should just chill out! This kind of medicine is rampant across the country.

With a lawyer-driven, sue-first mentality, doctors are afraid of malpractice. Depending on where the doctors live and what specialty they practice, annual malpractice insurance coverage is between $10,000 and $150,000. If a doctor loses their malpractice insurance, they cannot practice medicine. So you can see the dilemma. The better rapport the physician has with the patient, the less likely the doctor will be sued.

After the ER visit, patients are usually quite glad they had all the testing until they receive the bill. I would love to know the average cost per visit of the urgent care/ER versus the primary care visit for similar problems. Food for thought on the primary care provider vs. NP/PA choice. You and your family are flying from New York to London on Delta Airlines. You are getting ready for takeoff, and the flight attendant announces the pilot assistant will be flying you today. How do you feel?

Physician Burnout

If a physician tells you they have never experienced burnout in their career, they are lying! Burnout is defined as a combination of overwhelming exhaustion, depersonalization, detachment, a sense of ineffectiveness, and lack of accomplishment. Burnout can be defined differently by different people. Around four hundred physicians will die by suicide each year. Unless you are a physician, you cannot realize how overwhelming the occupation can be at times. Physicians make life-threatening decisions or perform operations daily.

If doctors begin medical school right after college, they will range from thirty to thirty-five years old when they can begin their practice. Most doctors will be over $200,000 in debt! And as mentioned, doctors then get the privilege of paying anywhere between $10,000 and $150,000 in malpractice insurance yearly—just so they can work every day! It is one of the few occupations that is highly scrutinized. They cannot make any mistakes, or they will have lawyers on their backs.

Managing a practice; dealing with insurance companies, patients, families, and pharmacies; using EMR; facing a lack of respect; autonomy control; working long hours, and being underappreciated all contribute to stress and burnout. It is hoped that one finds a wonderful significant other, a supportive family and a group of friends, and an outlet for stress.

I hope to give doctors a few suggestions to avoid or lessen burnout. Each day has only twenty-four hours, and no one is Superman. Time management is critical in any occupation.

First and foremost is family. I am sure no one on their deathbed wished they had worked harder! I tried to eliminate guilt and regret by attending or coaching my children in all of their endeavors. I can count on one hand the events I missed because of work. Make it a priority, and you will treasure all the moments.

I planned a date night with my wife once a week. We were cautious with our first-born child and always had family take care of him, but with the second and third kid, we left our Labrador Retriever to babysit!

You must take your allotted vacation time, a total of at least one month annually. You always need a light at the end of the tunnel to recharge the battery. Everyone needs an outlet or escape that does not include your family or work. Try golf, fishing, boating, knitting, join a book or card club, reading, exercising, or yoga, something where the mind can go elsewhere. Do not have your cell phone on during those activities.

If you find apathy setting in, you are drinking too much alcohol or eating too much, or you aren't enjoying your regular activities of daily living, do not be proud: Seek appropriate help.

Most doctors are driven, Type A personalities and are cut from the same cloth. When you finally finish your training and set up your practice, try to avoid the temptation to overdo it. You don't need the largest house, most expensive car or boat, or a country club membership as soon as you get your first paycheck. Try to live within your means, save money with each paycheck, and start a college education fund as soon as the children are born. Whatever lifestyle you choose will be obtainable with the amount of money physicians are paid.

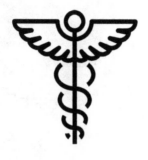

SECTION II

Medical Conditions

Chapter 1

Abdominal Pain

A bdominal pain is a complaint I hear every day. Obtaining a thorough history is the key to diagnosis along with just observing the patient. Does the patient appear toxic or describe the pain with a smile on their face? Is pain acute or chronic? Which side of the abdomen is the pain located? What makes the pain worse or better? What are the associated symptoms? Was there any trauma, recent surgery, or a rash? After the physical exam, I should have a pretty good idea of what the diagnosis is. I may want lab work, an ultrasound, or a CT scan, or I may refer the patient to the emergency room if deemed necessary. I will discuss a few of the common acute and chronic abdominal problems but refer to GERD in another section.

Acute Abdominal Pain

I refer to acute abdominal pain as symptoms and signs of such severity that it may require surgical intervention.

I am always concerned that I never miss these diagnoses. When I was just starting in private practice, I suspected a patient had acute appendicitis. I called a veteran surgeon and explained the situation, and he asked me what I wanted to do. I told him an ultrasound or CT scan of the abdomen, and he asked me why I would want that. He told me to trust my hands, the history, and the physical exam to make the diagnosis. Do not rely on technology! I have never forgotten those words of advice.

Acute Cholecystitis

Millions of people may have gallstones and do not even know it. Gallstones classically present with stomach or right upper quadrant abdominal pain an hour after a fatty meal and may radiate to the right shoulder blade. When a patient complains of acute onset of severe and steady pain in the stomach or right upper quadrant, and it's associated with fever, nausea, or vomiting, this could be cholecystitis. Murphy's sign on a physical exam is when the right upper quadrant is deeply palpated and causes the patient to quit breathing. These patients will be sent to the emergency room.

Acute Pancreatitis

Eighty percent of the time, acute pancreatitis is caused by alcohol abuse and gallstones. Eighty percent of patients will have a mild disease, but 20 percent will have severe symptoms. Patients experience severe diffuse abdominal pain, which may radiate to the back and include nausea, vomiting, fevers, shortness of breath, and jaundice (looking yellow). If the patient appears toxic, I will send them to the emergency room. If I am suspicious of the disease and the patient does not appear too ill and vital signs are normal, I will check amylase, lipase, complete blood count, and liver enzymes and order an ultrasound of the abdomen. I will send them home on a clear liquid diet and tell them to call me if symptoms become worse.

Acute Appendicitis

Acute appendicitis can appear at any age. Pain is usually in the right lower quadrant of the abdomen, but it can be in the mid or lower abdomen. Pain is accompanied with a fever, nausea, vomiting, and decreased appetite. Pain is usually worse with movement. On physical exam, I rely on rebound tenderness to determine if this is a surgical condition. When I push on the abdomen and let go, did the pain get worse? If the pain is worse when I let go, this is rebound tenderness. I will call my favorite surgeon and instruct them to go to the emergency room.

Acute Diverticulitis

Acute diverticulitis has fooled me on several occasions. It just never follows the classic symptoms (ha ha). As we all age and consume the usual American diet, the bowel wall weakens, causing pouches—like chuck holes in the road—called diverticula. Diverticula can get infected and patients may or may not have a fever, diarrhea, or abdominal pain in the left lower quadrant or right lower quadrant of the abdomen. Diverticula can rupture causing sepsis or free air in the abdomen. Fistula can occur—a connection/tunnel from the colon to the bladder—and you can have stool in the urine. One patient told me, "My penis is farting!" This is true because air is getting in the bladder. If diverticulitis is suspected in a healthy patient who does not appear toxic, and they have a normal physical exam except for tenderness, I will send them home with two antibiotics, Ciprofloxacin and Flagyl, a clear liquid diet, and instructions to go to the emergency room if they get worse. Alcohol cannot be consumed while on Flagyl, or you will puke your brains out. If the patient appears toxic, is dehydrated, has a fever, or has an elevated heart rate, I will have them go to the emergency room.

Chronic Abdominal Pain

Inflammatory Bowel Disease

Inflammatory bowel disease (IBD) is inflammation of the gastrointestinal tract. It is divided into ulcerative colitis and Crohn's disease. There are subtle differences between the two, but for the sake of discussion, they will be referred to as IBD. Common symptoms are abdominal pain, weight loss, fever or no fever, incontinence of stool, and diarrhea may or may not be bloody. Some patients have no diarrhea. Ten percent of patients have extra intestinal manifestations, meaning symptoms that do not involve the gastrointestinal tract. One of my patient's only problems was elevated liver enzymes. Other manifestations can be sacroiliitis, mouth sores, arthritis, eye redness or pain, and skin disease. If IBD is suspected, a complete blood count, metabolic panel, total protein, and C-reactive protein are checked. A GI specialist will perform a colonoscopy with biopsies to confirm the diagnosis. If the diagnosis is confirmed, I do not feel comfortable treating these patients as treatment options do evolve and specialists should be in charge.

Irritable Bowel Syndrome

Irritable bowel syndrome (IBS) is abdominal pain associated with diarrhea, constipation, or alternating between the two. IBS is more common in women and in younger adults. The cause is unknown, and it is a diagnosis of exclusion. This means that doctors feel that no other possible disease is causing these symptoms. A patient may have abdominal pain or discomfort relieved with a bowel movement, change of frequency or form of stool, or loose or watery stools. If a patient has anemia, weight loss, a family history of colon cancer, or celiac disease, the doctor should rule out these disorders prior to making the diagnosis of IBS.

Treatment for IBS with constipation is increased hydration, fiber, and laxatives as needed. Medication is required most of the time. Patients have good success with Linzess. Linzess is taken once a day, usually has good insurance coverage, and comes in three different doses. Diarrhea is a side effect. Treatment of IBS with diarrhea begins with increased hydration, fiber, and Imodium as needed.

If patients are having increased abdominal pain, Bentyl is helpful. Viberzi is taken twice a day but cannot be used if patients have had their gallbladder removed or have a history of pancreatitis and alcoholism. I have not used Xifaxan as much, secondary to the cost and poor insurance coverage. Xifaxan's advantage is it is only taken three times a day for two weeks and repeated every six months.

Sometimes none of the medications are helpful. I have found that stress and anxiety, even when patients go on vacation, out to eat, or to the mall, can exacerbate their symptoms. Patients have had success with SSRIs like Zoloft or the old anti-depression medicine Elavil to help prevent exacerbation.

Chapter 2

Alcoholism

Everyone needs to remember that alcoholism is a disease. Patients are genetically predisposed to developing alcoholism. Alcoholism has no favorites as it affects all ages, races, and socioeconomic groups. An alcoholic once told me he was not an alcoholic because he drank too much alcohol; it was because he could never have enough alcohol! A definition of alcoholism is having four drinks a day or more than fourteen drinks in a week. Alcoholics have a strong desire or urge for alcohol. They cannot control their use of alcohol even if it causes a DUI, job loss, divorce, prison, or, in the end, death.

I use the CAGE screening for alcohol abuse:

C = Have you ever felt you should *Cut down on your drinking?*
A = Have people *Annoyed you* by criticizing your drinking?

G = Have you ever felt *Guilty about your drinking?*
E = *Have* you ever had an *Eye-opener* drink first thing in the morning to get rid of a hangover?

If the answer is yes to any of the above, the patient most likely has a problem.

Alcohol abuse can lead to hypertension, stroke, peptic ulcers, cirrhosis, bone marrow toxicity, pancreatitis, and multiple cancers. Patients are usually aware of the risks, just as with smoking, and continue to consume alcohol until they hit rock bottom. Rock bottom is different for every individual. Alcoholics cannot stop drinking alcohol until they want to stop for themselves. Family, friends, and coworkers are all affected. Al-Anon support groups teach the family and friends of alcoholics never to forget the Three Cs: You did not Cause it. You cannot Control it. You cannot Cure it.

Treatment is multifactorial once the patient admits the problem. I never had good luck with medications, such as Antabuse, when treating patients. Alcoholics Anonymous (AA) is a tremendous program as it teaches the Twelve-Step program and is very spiritual. Veterans of AA have heard, seen, and experienced it all, and there is no shame. You cannot fool anyone because members of the group will call you out. The group will become like family. AA members have true empathy, not sympathy. Even when the alcoholic falls off the wagon, which many do, other members urge that person to keep on trying—keep attending meetings and take it one day at a time! Your life will be significantly better!

All significant others will go through the same behavioral process when dealing with an alcoholic. It goes from denial to enabling and anger to finally acceptance. I encourage significant others to attend Al-Anon as it is a place of solace. Al-Anon is another group where you can let your guard down, be truthful without experiencing judgment, learn coping mechanisms, and learn from the veterans of the group. You will become aware and learn of the deception the alcoholics have successfully used to continue drinking and justify it. Trust must be earned. When relapses occur, tough love may be the best love you have ever given. Family counseling is recommended, either through church or family counseling. Everyone should turn to their higher power for guidance.